CONTENTS

Section I

ASSESSMENT/TREATMENT GUIDELINES

QUICK REFERENCE FOR

Clinical Nursing

Second Edition

June M. Thompson, RN, DrPH
Director of Nursing Research, Education, and Standards
University Hospital
University of New Mexico Health Sciences Center
Albuquerque, New Mexico

with 15 illustrations

The author and publisher have made a conscientious effort to ensure that the drug information and recommended dosages in this book are accurate and in accord with accepted standards at the time of publication. However, pharmacology is a rapidly changing science, so readers are advised to check the package insert provided by the manufacturer before administering any drug.

Mosby Year Book

St. Louis Baltimore Boston Chicago London Philadelphia Sydney Toronto

Mosby
Dedicated to Publishing Excellence

Vice President and Publisher: Nancy L. Coon
Senior Editor: Sally Schrefer
Developmental Editor: Gail Brower

SECOND EDITION

Printed in the United States of America
Composition by The Clarinda Co.
Lithography by The Clarinda Co.
Printing/binding by Mulligan Printing Co.

Mosby–Year Book, Inc.
11830 Westline Industrial Drive
St. Louis, Missouri 63146

International Standard Book Number 0-8151-3721-4

97 98 99 00 CL/PC 9 8 7 6 5 4 3 2 1

SECTION I ASSESSMENT/TREATMENT GUIDELINES

GENERAL ASSESSMENT

Adult Preventive Care Guidelines (ANA)

Checkup visits with a physician or other health care provider are important for good health. Most authorities recommend these visits every 1 to 3 years until age 65 and yearly thereafter. Each individual should speak with a physician or other health care provider about the proper schedule of checkup visits.

Tests

Blood pressure—Every 2 years, beginning age 18
Height and weight—Periodically
Cholesterol—Every 5 years, beginning age 35 (age 18*)
Hearing—Every 5 years, beginning age 35 (age 18*)
Mammography—Periodically, beginning age 65
Pap smear (women)—Every 1 to 2 years, beginning age 50 (age 40*)
Prostate-specific antigen (men)—Yearly, beginning age 50*
Sigmoidoscopy—Every 3 to 5 years*
Stool occult blood—Yearly*
Urinalysis—Periodically*

Exams

Dental—Yearly, from age 18
Vision/glaucoma—Every 2 to 4 years, beginning age 40*; every 2 years, beginning age 60

---

*Recommended by some major authorities.

Breast (women)—Every 1 to 3 years, beginning age 18*; yearly beginning age 40

Exams for cancer (thyroid, mouth, skin, ovaries, testicles, lymph nodes, rectum [40+], prostate[men 50+])—Every 3 years, beginning age 18*; yearly after age 40*

Immunizations

Tetanus-diphtheria—Every 10 years, beginning age 18
Pneumococcal—Once at age 65
Influenza—Yearly after age 65

Health guidance

Smoking, alcohol and drugs, sexual behavior, AIDS, nutrition, physical activity, violence and guns, family planning, injuries, occupational health, folate (women 12-45), *aspirin* (men 40+), *estrogen* (women 45+)—Periodically

Please note: Recommended intervals for each type of preventive care may vary among authorities. Time intervals given are recommended by all major authorities unless indicated otherwise. Individuals with special risk factors may need more frequent and additional types of preventive care. Some examples:

Risk factor	Preventive service(s) needed
Diabetes	Eye, foot examinations, urine test
Drug abuse	AIDS, TB test, hepatitis immunization

Data from American Nurses Association (ANA): *Put Prevention into Practice (PPIP)*, Waldorf, Maryland, 1995, American Nurses Publishing.
*Recommended by some major authorities.

Alcoholism	Influenza, pneumococcal immunizations, TB test
Overweight	Blood sugar test
Homeless, recent refugee or immigrant	TB test
High-risk sexual behavior	AIDS, syphilis, gonorrhea, chlamydia tests

Children Preventive Care Guidelines (ANA)

Checkup visits are important for a child's health. Some authorities recommend these visits at the following ages: 2 to 4 weeks; 2, 4, 6, 9, 12, 15, and 18 months; and 2, 3, 4, 5, 6, 8, 10, 12, 14, 16, and 18 years. A child's physician or other health care provider will discuss the individual needs of the child. At checkup visits, a child may receive a physical examination and the types of preventive care shown below.

Tests

Newborn screening—At birth
Head size—Birth to 2 years
Height and weight—Birth to 18 years
Blood pressure—3 to 18 years
Anemia—6 to 12 months; 2 to 3 years, 8 to 9 years, and 18 years*
Lead—1 to 3 years*
Urinalysis—Birth to 1 year, 2 to 3 years, 8 to 9 years, 18 years*
Tuberculosis—1 to 2 years, 4 to 5 years, 14 to 15 years*
Hearing—4 to 6 years, 12 to 13 years, 18 years*
Vision—3 to 4 years; 4 to 7 years, 8 to 9 years, 12 to 13 years, 14 to 15 years, 18 years*

Exams

Eye—Birth to 1 year, 3 to 4 years; 5 to 6 years*
Dental—1 to 3½ years*; 3½ years to 18 years

Immunizations

Hepatitis B (HBV)—3 times, birth to 18 months
Polio (OPV)—3 times, 2 to 9 months; once, 4 to 6 years
Haemophilus influenzae (Hib)—3 or 4 times, 2 to 18 months
Diphtheria, tetanus, pertussis (DTP, Td)—4 times, 2 to 18 months; once, 4 to 6 years
Measles, mumps, rubella (MMR)—Once, 16 to 18 month; once, 4 to 6 years*; once, 11 to 12 years (if not given at 4-6 years)*
Chickenpox (VZV)—Once, 12 to 18 months

Health guidance

Development, nutrition, oral health, physical activity, injuries and poisons, sun exposure, smoking, alcohol and drugs, AIDS, sexual behavior, family planning—As appropriate for age

Please note: Children with special risk factors may need more frequent and additional types of preventive care. Some examples:

Risk factor	**Preventive service(s) needed**
Exposure to TB	TB test
Sexually active	Pap test (females); syphilis, gonorrhea, chlamydia tests
High-risk sexual behavior	AIDS test, hepatitis immunization
Drug abuse	AIDS test, TB test, hepatitis immunication

---

*Recommended by some major authorities.
Data from American Nurses Association (ANA): *Put Prevention into Practice (PPIP)*, Waldorf, Maryland, 1995, American Nurses Publishing.
*Recommended by some major authorities.

Vital Signs

Vital Sign Ranges

	Pulse	Respirations	Blood Pressure
Newborn	120 to 160	30 to 50	60 to 96/30 to 62 mm Hg
Toddlers (1-3 years)	90 to 140	20 to 30	78 to 112/48 to 78 mm Hg
Preschool (4-6 years)	80 to 110	18 to 26	78 to 112/50 to 82 mm Hg
School age (7-11 years)	75 to 110	16 to 22	85 to 114/52 to 85 mm Hg
Adolescent (12-16 years)	60 to 100	14 to 20	94 to 136/58 to 88 mm Hg
Adult	60 to 110	12 to 20	100 to 140/60 to 90 mm Hg

Data from Cannobbio,[7] Wong,[25] Thompson and Wilson.[23]

ANALYSIS OF A SYMPTOM

Location—Where are the symptoms?

- Is the location in a specific area? Vague and generalized? Does symptom radiate?

Quality—Describe the characteristics of the symptom.

- Describe the sensation: stabbing, dull, aching, throbbing, nagging, sharp, squeezing, itching.
- Describe the drainage: color, texture, composition, appearance, and odor.
- Was the onset slow? Abrupt? Noticeable to others?
- Was the symptom intermittent or continuous?
- How has symptom interrupted your life (e.g., sleeping, eating, working, activities at home or school)?

Quantity—Describe the severity of the symptom.

- Describe the size, extent, number, or amount (e.g., of lesion, rash, blister, discharge).
- Was the symptom so severe that it interrupted your activities?
- On a scale of 1 to 10, with 10 being most severe, how would you rate your symptom?

Chronology—When did the symptom start?

- Ask specific date, time, day of the week.
- How many times a day, week, month did symptom occur?
- How did client feel in between episodes of the symptom?

Setting—Where are you when the symptom occurs?

- Does anyone else with whom you have been in contact have a similar symptom?
- Are there psychologic or physical factors in the environment that may be causing the symptom (e.g., stress or smoke or chemicals)?

Associated manifestations—Do other symptoms occur at the same time?

- What effect does the symptom have on body function? activities? appetite?

Alleviating factors

- What home remedies have you tried?
- What medications have you tried (over-the-counter and prescription)?
- Are there certain body positions that relieve symptom?

Aggravating factors

- Is symptom associated with an activity (e.g., walking, climbing stairs, eating, a body position)?

Conceptual Model of Pain

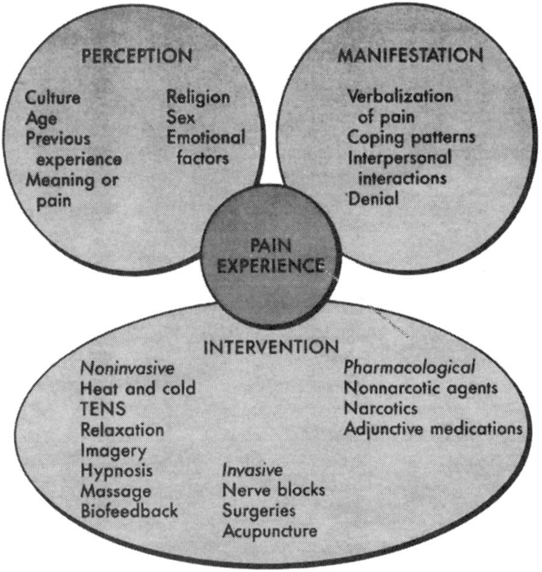

Three aspects of pain: perception, manifestation, and intervention. *Perception* includes factors that affect one's perception of pain such as culture, religion, age, gender, past experience, and emotional factors such as anxiety. *Manifestation* shows that the most important factor in this aspect of pain is the patient's verbalization, or statement, of his pain, or the patient's denial of his pain. *Intervention* divides methods of intervention into three types (noninvasive, invasive, and pharmacological). (From Beare, Myers.[4])

Examples of Nonpharmacologic Interventions for Pain

Cognitive-Behavioral

- Education/instruction
- Relaxation
- Imagery
- Music distraction
- Biofeedback

Physical Agents

- Applications of heat or cold
- Massage, exercise, and immobilization
- Transcutaneous electrical nerve stimulation

Jaw Relaxation Instructions

- Let your lower jaw drop slightly, as though you were starting a small yawn.
- Keep your tongue quiet and resting on the bottom of your mouth.
- Let your lips get soft.
- Breathe slowly, evenly, and rhythmically: inhale, exhale, and rest.
- Allow yourself to stop forming words with your lips and stop thinking in words.

Reprinted with permission. McCaffery, M. and Beebe, A. (1989). *Pain: Clinical manual for nursing practice*. St. Louis: Mosby.

Pain Assessment Tools

Pain Intensity Scales

Simple Descriptive Pain Intensity Scale*

No pain	Mild pain	Moderate pain	Severe pain	Very severe pain	Worse possible pain

0 to 10 Numeric Pain Intensity Scale*

0	1	2	3	4	5	6	7	8	9	10

Pain Distress Scales

Simple Descriptive Pain Distress Scale*

None	Annoying	Uncomfortable	Dreadful	Horrible	Agonizing

0 to 10 Numeric Pain Distress Scale*

0	1	2	3	4	5	6	7	8	9	10

*If used as a graphic rating scale, a 10 cm baseline is recommended.

Reference: AHCPR Pain Management Clinical Practice Guideline.[1]

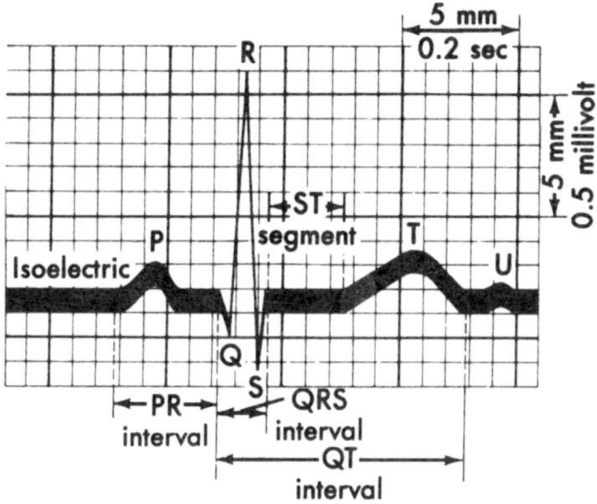

Cardiac Cycle

The cardiac cycle includes the following waveforms and time intervals:

P wave—The electrical activity associated with the sinus node impulse and its depolarization of the atria

PR interval—The time the impulse takes to travel through the atria to the A-V node, the bundle of His and bundle branches, and the ventricles; normal duration is 0.12 to 0.20 second

Classifications of Hypertension

Types of Hypertension According to Cause

Primary (essential, idiopathic)—No known etiology or evident cause
Secondary—Develops secondary to an identifiable mechanism

Isolated systolic hypertension—Systolic pressure ≥ 160 mm Hg and normal diastolic pressure usually associated with age

Early primary hypertension—A pressure higher than normotensive

Refractory or resistant—Failure to achieve normotensive diastolic pressure < 140/90 mm Hg on a rational triple drug regimen in close to maximal doses

Pregnancy-induced hypertension—An increase in BP of 15 mm Hg above first trimester levels during pregnancy

White coat hypertension—Elevated blood pressure at clinic visits but normal daytime ambulatory pressures

Types of Hypertension According to Severity

Mild—A diastolic pressure of 90 to 104 mm Hg

Moderate—A diastolic pressure of 104 to 114 mm Hg

Severe—A diastolic pressure of more than 115 mm Hg

Malignant—A syndrome of encephalopathy and papilledema with hypertension

Borderline—Pressures that occasionally go up to the mild range

---

From Beare, Myers.[4]

Types of Innocent Murmurs

Vibratory systolic murmur
Pulmonic ejection systolic murmur
Aortic midsystolic murmur
Supraclavicular systolic murmur
Systolic or continuous mammary soufflé
Venous hum

From Canobbio.7

Grading of Cardiac Murmurs

Classification	Description
Grade I	Soft, barely audible in quiet room
Grade II	Quiet but clearly audible
Grade III	Moderately loud, without thrill
Grade IV	Loud, associated with thrill
Grade V	Very loud, thrill easily palpable
Grade VI	Very loud, audible with stethoscope off the chest, thrill palpable and visible

From Canobbio.[7]

Pitting Edema Scale

Scale	Degree	Response
1+ Trace	Slight	Rapid
2+ Mild	0–0.6 cm (0-¼ in)	10-15 seconds
3+ Moderate	0.6-1.3 cm (¼-½ in)	1-2 minutes
4+ Severe	1.3-2.5 cm (½-1 in)	2-5 minutes

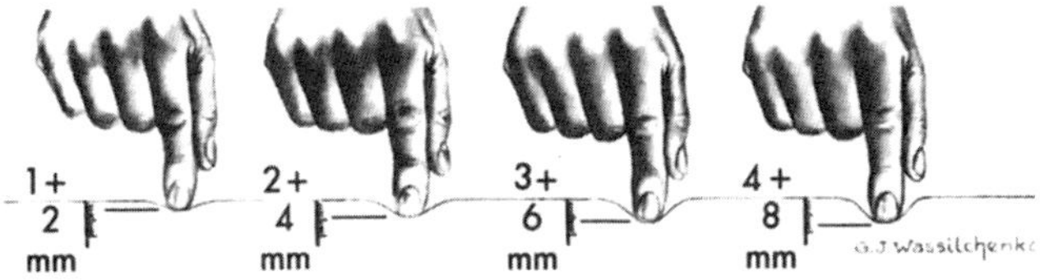

From Canobbio.[7]

Auscultation of the Heart

A systematic approach is needed for this assessment. Some examiners begin at the apex and proceed upward toward the base of the heart, while others begin at the base and proceed downward toward the apex. The sequence is irrelevant as long as the assessment is systematic. Listen first with the diaphragm to hear high-pitched sounds, then with the bell to hear low-pitched sounds.

- When auscultating from base to apex, begin at the second intercostal space (ICS). Locate this ICS by palpating the right sternoclavicular joint (where the left clavicle joins the sternum.)
- Palpate the first rib and then move down to palpate the space between the first and second ribs; this is the first ICS.
- Continue palpating downward to the space between the second and third ribs. This is the second ICS at the right sternal border (RSB), the auscultatory site for the aortic value area. This is not the anatomic site of the aortic valve, but the site on the chest wall where sounds produced by the valves are heard best.
- Moving to the left side of the sternum at the second ICS, the area for auscultating the pulmonic valve area is found.
- Remaining at the LSB, move the stethoscope down to the third ICS, which is called Erb's point, an area to which pulmonic or aortic sounds frequently radiate. The fourth ICS, LSB is over the tricuspid valve area.
- At the fifth ICS, move the stethoscope laterally to the left midclavicular line, where the mitral valve area is located.

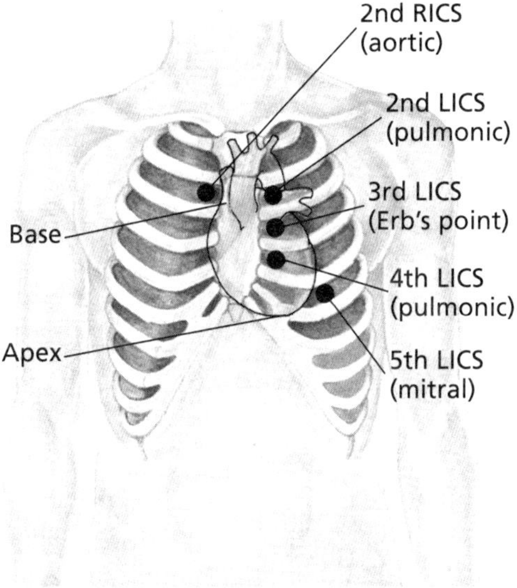

From Thompson/Wilson.[24]

RESPIRATORY
Patterns of Respiration

Pattern	Description	Associated Conditions
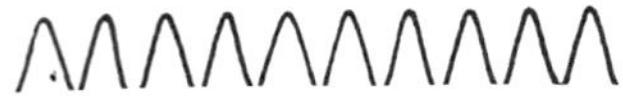	Normal: smooth and even at a rate of 12-20/min	
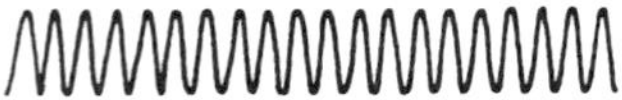	Tachypnea: shallow breathing at a rate of >20/min	Anxiety, pain, massive liver enlargement, abdominal ascites
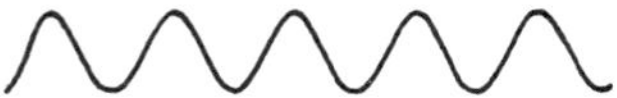	Bradypnea: <12/min	Neurogenic disorders, electrolyte imbalance, infection, protective response to pain or pleurisy or other discomfort aggravated by breathing
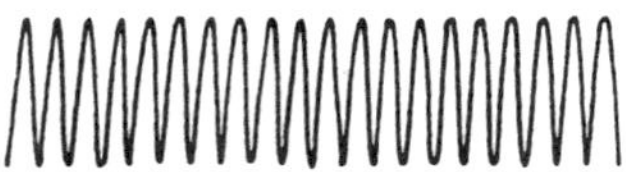	Hyperpnea or hyperventilation: deep breathing at a rate of >20/min	Exercise, acute anxiety, panic reactions, metabolic disorders
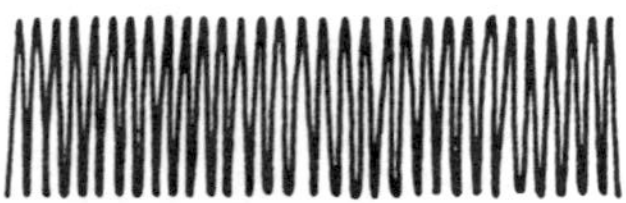	Kussmaul: fast (>20/min), deep, sighing breaths without pauses; labored breathing	Renal failure, metabolic acidosis

Pattern	Description	Associated Conditions
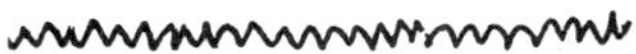	Central neurogenic hyperventilation: hyperpnea over a sustained period	Lesions in lower midbrain or upper pons, often secondary to transtentorial herniation
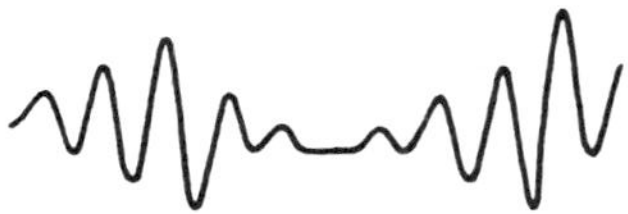	Cheyne-Stokes: alternating hyperpnea and apnea	In adults, bilateral lesions in cerebral hemisphere, basal ganglia, midbrain, pons, or cerebellum. In infants this pattern is normal
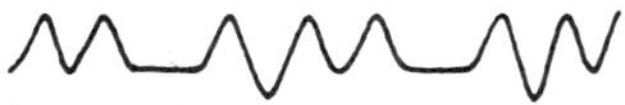	Biot's or cluster: disorganized sequence of breaths with irregular periods of apnea	Lesions of lower pons or upper medulla
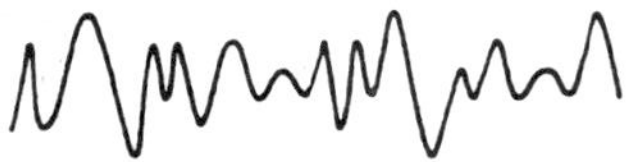	Ataxic breathing: irregular breathing patterns with both deep and shallow breaths occurring randomly	Lesions of medulla

From Thompson/Wilson.[24]

Blood Gas Values and Interpretation

Blood Gases: Normal Values

Arterial		Venous
7.35-7.45	pH	7.31-7.41
80-100 mm Hg	paO_2*	30-40 mm Hg
35-45 mm Hg	pCo_2	41-51 mm Hg
21-25 mEq/L	HCO_3	22-29 mEq/L
95%-99%	O_2 sat	60%-85%

*In a patient >60 years old, PaO_2 is equal to 80 mm Hg minus 1 mm Hg for every year over 60. Expected PaO_2 can be determined by multiplying the FiO_2 by 5.

Interpreting ABGs

1. Check pH
   - ↑ = Alkalosis
   - ↓ = Acidosis
   - nl = No imbalance
2. Check pCo_2
   - ↑ = CO_2 retention (hypoventilation); respiratory acidosis or compensatory for metabolic alkalosis
   - ↓ = CO_2 blown off (hyperventilation); respiratory alkalosis or compensating for metabolic acidosis
   - nl = No imbalance of respiratory component
3. Check HCO_3
   - ↑ = Nonvolatile acid is lost; HCO_3 gained (metabolic alkalosis or compensating for respiratory acidosis)
   - ↓ = Nonvolatile acid is added; HCO_3 is lost (metabolic acidosis or compensating for respiratory alkalosis)
4. Determine imbalance
5. Determine if compensation exists

Normal values for arterial blood gases and abnormal values in uncompensated acid-base disturbances

Acid-base disturbance	pH	PCo_2 mm Hg	HCO-mEq/L	Common Cause
None (normal values)	7.35-7.45	35-45	22-26	
Respiratory acidosis	↓	↑	Normal	Respiratory depression
				Pulmonary disease
Respiratory alkalosis	↑	↓	Normal	Hyperventilation
Metabolic acidosis	↓	Normal	↓	Diabetes, shock, renal failure
Metabolic alkalosis	↑	Normal	↑	Sodium bicarbonate overdose
				Prolonged vomiting
				Nasogastric drainage

From Pagana and Pagana.[18]

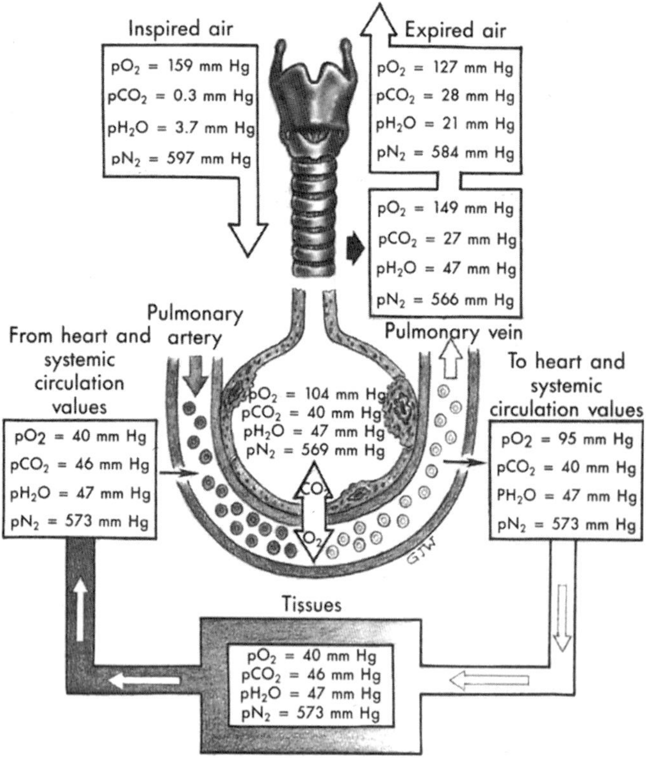

Partial pressure of respiratory gases in normal respiration.

Oxyhemoglobin Dissociation Curve

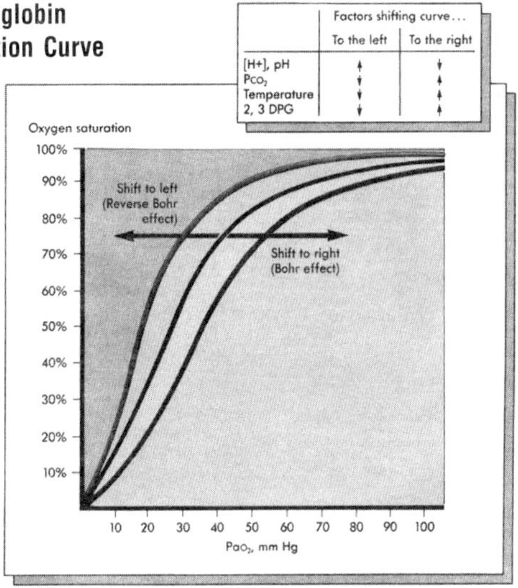

	Factors shifting curve...	
	To the left	To the right
[H+], pH	↑	↓
PCO_2	↓	↑
Temperature	↓	↑
2, 3 DPG	↓	↑

A *shift to the right* indicates that hemoglobin's intrinsic ability to hold on to oxygen has weakened and higher partial pressures are needed for binding. O_2 escapes hemoglobin more easily and is more available to tissues. This shift is produced by decreased pH, increased $PaCO_2$, and increased temperature or by prolonged hypoxia. *Normal curve* occurring at blood pH 7.4, normal $PaCO_2$, and body temperature at 37°C. A *shift to the left* indicates hemoglobin and oxygen are bound too tightly and, although less pressure is needed for binding, the molecules separate with difficulty at the cellular level. O_2 is less available to tissues. This shift is produced by increased pH, decreased $PaCO_2$, and decrease in temperature. It can also occur with prolonged hypoxia in which 2, 3-diphosphoglycerate (DPG) increases inside red blood cells. (From Wilson.[21])

Contraindications and Cautions for Oxygen Therapy

1. Oxygen-induced hypoventilation: when the arterial carbon dioxide tension is greater than 50 mm Hg, the risk of oxygen-induced hypoventilation increases. It is therefore advised, especially for patients with chronic lung diseases, to maintain oxygen therapy so the arterial oxygen tension remains about 50 to 60 mm Hg.

   To prevent this problem use low concentrations of oxygen if the patient is not mechanically ventilated. Observe ventilatory pattern and quality.

2. Atelectasis: the collapse of alveoli may occur secondary to high concentrations of oxygen in inspired air, which causes malfunctioning pulmonary surfactant.

   To prevent this complication, if possible limit the duration of 100% inspired oxygen to no more than 20 minutes; maintain patient airway; sigh the patient if on a ventilator; and provide high tidal volumes.

3. Oxygen toxicity: the lungs can normally handle oxygen concentrations of 21%. Although it is not clear exactly what fractional inspired oxygen (FIO_2) percent causes oxygen toxicity, it is most probable that an FIO_2 of over 50% administered for longer than 24 hours increases the risk.

Weaning from the Ventilator

Physiologic Guidelines

1. Vital capacity at least 10 to 15 ml/kg body weight
2. Alveolar-arterial oxygen tension difference (PAO_2–PaO_2) measured with patient receiving 100% oxygen should be less than 300 to 500 mm Hg
3. Maximum inspiratory force greater than 20 cm H_2O
4. Tidal volume greater than 5 ml/kg
5. Resting minute ventilation greater than 10 L/minute
6. $PaCO_2$ within stable range
7. PaO_2 greater than 70 to 80 mm Hg on 0.5 FIO_2
8. PaO_2 on 100% oxygen greater than 300 mm Hg
9. Shunt fraction less than 15%

If the patient is not completely ready to be weaned from the ventilator, intermittent mandatory ventilation (IMV) or intermittent demand ventilation (IDV) may be initiated.

Cranial Nerves and their Function

Cranial Nerves	Function
Olfactory (I)	Sensory: smell reception and interpretation
Optic (II)	Sensory: visual acuity and visual fields
Oculomotor (III)	Motor: raise eyelids, most extraocular movements
	Parasympathetic: pupillary constriction, change lens shape
Trochlear (IV)	Motor: downward, inward eye movement
Trigeminal (V)	Motor: jaw opening and clenching, chewing and mastication
	Sensory: sensation to cornea, iris, lacrimal glands, conjunctiva eyelids, forehead, nose, nasal and mouth mucosa, teeth, tongue, ear, facial skin
Abducens (VI)	Motor: lateral eye movement
Facial (VII)	Motor: movement of facial expression muscles except jaw, close eyes, labial speech sounds (b, m, w, and rounded vowels)
	Sensory: taste—anterior two thirds of tongue, sensation to pharynx
	Parasympathetic: secretion of saliva and tears
Acoustic (VIII)	Sensory: hearing and equilibrium

Cranial Nerves and their Function—cont'd

Cranial Nerves	Function
Glossopharyngeal (IX)	Motor: voluntary muscles for swallowing and phonation
	Sensory: sensation of nasopharynx, gag reflex, taste—posterior one third of tongue
	Parasympathetic: secretion of salivary glands, carotid reflex
Vagus (X)	Motor: voluntary muscles of phonation (guttural speech sounds) and swallowing
	Sensory: sensation behind ear and part of external ear canal
	Parasympathetic: secretion of digestive enzymes; peristalsis; carotid reflex; involuntary action of heart, lungs, and digestive tract
Spinal accessory (XI)	Motor: turn head, shrug shoulders, some actions for phonation
Hypoglossal (XII)	Motor: tongue movement for speech sound articulation (l, t, n) and swallowing

From Seidel et al.[20]

Spinal Nerves

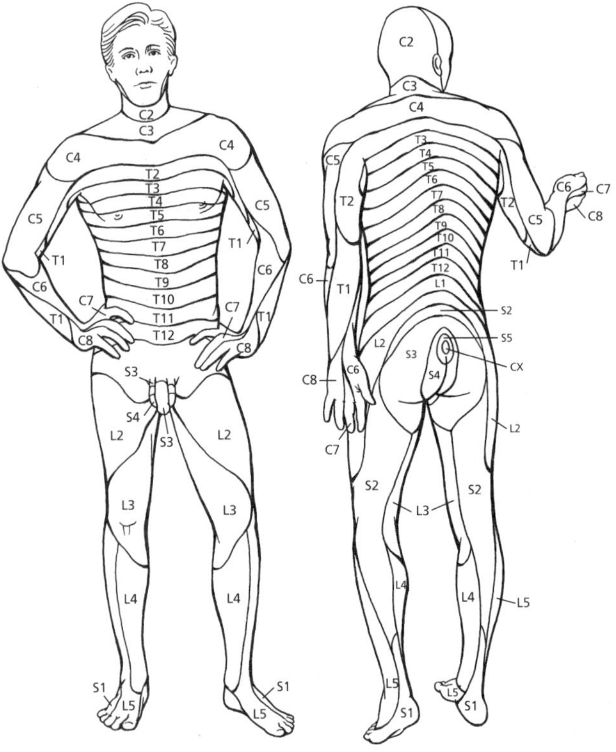

From Seeley, Stephens, Tate.[21]

Functional Goals in Spinal Cord Lesions

Spinal cord level	Muscle function	Functional goals
C3–C4	Neck control Scapular elevators	Manipulate electric wheelchair with mouth stick Limited self-feeding with ball bearing feeders
C5	Fair to good shoulder control Good elbow flexion	Dress upper trunk Turn self in bed with arm slings Propel wheelchair with handrim projections Self-feeding with handsplints Assist getting to and from bed
C6	Good shoulder control Wrist extension Supinators	Transfer from wheelchair to bed and car with minimal or no assistance Self-feeding with tenodesis hands Assist in getting to and from commode chair

Functional Goals in Spinal Cord Lesions—cont'd

Spinal cord level	Muscle function	Functional goals
C7	Weak shoulder depression Weak elbow extension Some hand function	Independent in transfer to bed, car, and toilet Total dressing independence Wheelchair without handrim projections Self-feeding with no assistive devices
C8–T4	Good to normal upper extremity muscle function	Wheelchair to floor and return Wheelchair up and down curb Wheelchair to tub and return
T5–L2	Partial to good trunk stability	Total wheelchair independence Limited ambulation with bilateral long leg braces and crutches
L3–L4	All trunk-pelvic stabilizers intact Hip flexors Adductors Quadriceps	Ambulation with short leg braces with or without crutches, depending on level
L5	Hip extensors, abductors, knee flexors, ankle control	No equipment needed if plantar flexion enough for push off at end of stance

From Beare, Myers.[4]

Muscle Function According to Level of Spinal Cord Injury

Spinal cord level	Level of function
C4 and above	Loss of all muscle function including respiratory function (usually fatal)
C5	Quadriplegia with poor respiratory functioning
C6-C8	Quadriplegia with sparing of some arm and hand muscles
T1-T3	Quadriplegia with loss of muscle function below nipple line
T4–T10	Paraplegia with some chest and trunk muscles intact
T11-L2	Paraplegia with muscles intact through upper thigh
L3-S1	Paraplegia with muscles of chest, trunk, thigh, and most of leg intact; loss of voluntary bowel and bladder control
S2-S4	Loss of voluntary bowel and bladder control

Neurovascular Checks

Parameter	Significance
Color of affected and surrounding tissues	Indicates adequacy of circulation; color should be pinkish, not pale or white. Injured tissues are usually paler than the contralateral tissues.
Temperature of affected tissue	Indicates circulatory adequacy or perfusion. Injured tissues are usually cooler than contralateral tissues.
Capillary refill of nails	Refill in 2-3 seconds indicates normal capillary perfusion. Initially, injured tissues may have normal refill, but gradual slowing may be noted with careful assessment; slowing to 4-6 seconds should be reported.
Edema	Presence indicates venous stasis. Injured tissues usually are noticeably more swollen than contralateral tissues.

Neurovascular Checks—cont'd

Parameter	Significance
Range of motion or movement of tissues	Indicates amount or degree of limitation(s) of movement. Injured tissues usually have decreased mobility (patient may hold the part to lessen pain).
Sensory functions (may not be diagnostic in newborn or very young baby)	Indicates pressure on nerves, noted by complaints of numbness, tingling, or "pins and needles" sensation.
Complaints of pain	Indicates injury, pressure, or trauma to tissues. Injured tissues usually are more painful than contralateral tissues.
Affected and unaffected tissues bilaterally	Indicates specific tissue involved when compared with other side.

From Mourad.[17]

Scale for Deep Tendon Reflexes

Test the five deep tendon reflexes (triceps, biceps, brachioradial, patellar and achilles) using a reflex hammer. Compare the reflexes bilaterally. Reflexes are graded on a scale of 0 to 4+ with 2+ being the expected findings. Findings are recorded as follows:

0 = No response

1+ = Sluggish or diminished

2+ = Active or expected response

3+ = Slightly hyperactive, more brisk than normal; not necessarily pathologic

4+ = Brisk, hyperactive with intermittent clonus associated with disease

---

From Thompson/Wilson.[24]

Pupil Scale (in Millimeters)

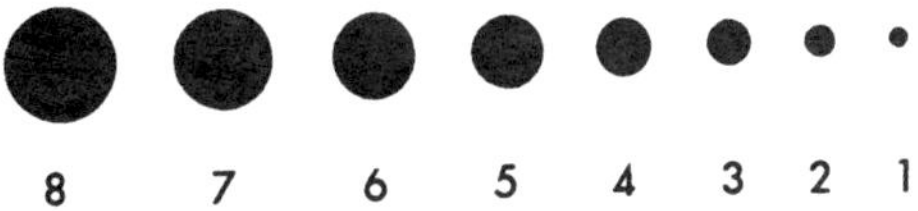

(From Madigan.[11])

Pediatric Coma Scale

	<2 years	>2 years	
Eye opening	Spontaneous	Spontaneous	4
	To voice	To voice	3
	To pain	To pain	2
	None	None	1
Verbal	Coos, babbles	Oriented	5
	Irritable, consolable	Confused	4
	Cries to pain, inconsolable	Inappropriate	3
	Moans to pain	Garbled	2
	None	None	1
Motor	Normal movements	Obeys commands	6
	Withdraws to touch	Localizes pain	5
	Withdraws to pain	Withdraws to pain	4
	Flexion	Flexion	3
	Extension	Extension	2
	Flaccid	Flaccid	1

(From Wong.[26])

Glasgow Coma Scale

Best eye-opening response	Spontaneously	4
	To verbal command	3
	To pain	2
	No response	1
Best verbal response	Oriented, converses	5
	Disoriented, converses	4
	Inappropriate words	3
	Incomprehensible sounds	2
	No response	1
Best motor response		
To verbal command	Obeys	6
To painful stimulus	Localizes pain	5
	Flexion-withdrawal	4
	Flexion-decorticate	3
	Extension-decerebrate	2
	No response	1
	TOTAL	(3-15)

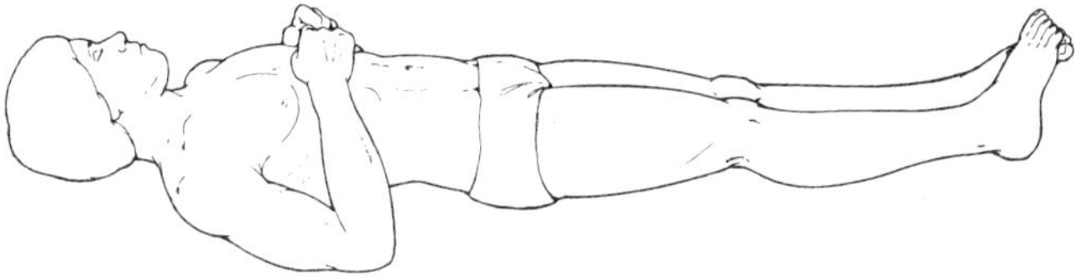

Decorticate Rigid flexion; upper arms held tightly to the sides of body; elbows, wrists, and fingers flexed; feet are plantar flexed, legs extended and internally rotated; may have fine tremors or intense stiffness

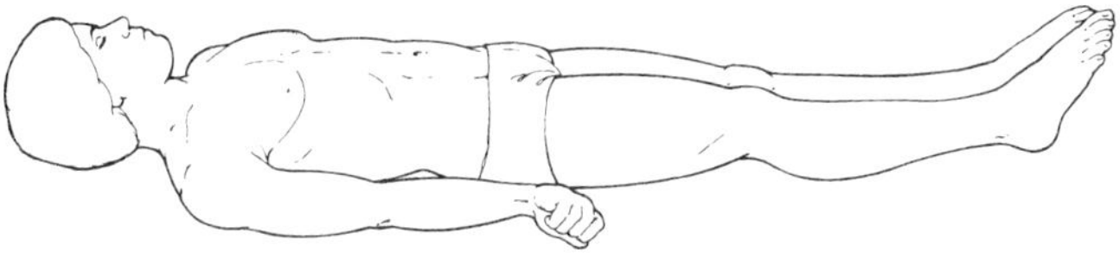

Decerebrate Rigid extension; arms fully extended; forearms pronated; wrists and fingers flexed; jaws clenched, neck extended, back may be arched; feet plantar flexed; may occur spontaneously, intermittently, or in response to a stimulus

From Thompson/Wilson.[24]

SKIN

Lesion Characteristics

- Note the **location and distribution** of the lesion. Is the lesion generalized over the entire body or section of the body, or is it localized to a specific area such as around the waist, under a piece of jewelry, or just in the hair?
- Describe the **color** of the lesion and describe how this lesion may be different in color from other lesions noted on the body (e.g., a mole or freckle). Has the patient noticed a change in the color of the lesion?
- What is the **pattern** of the lesion? Are the lesions clustered? Are they in a line? How does the patient describe the development of the pattern of the lesion?
- What are the **edges** of the lesion like? Is the edge of the lesion regular or irregular? Has the patient noticed a change in the shape of the lesion?
- Is the lesion **flat, raised, or sunken?**
- What is the current **size** of the lesion? Measure using a centimeter ruler. Has the patient noticed a change in the size of the lesion?
- What are the **characteristics** of the lesion? Is it hard, soft, or fluid-filled? If there is an exudate, what is the color of the drainage fluid? Does the exudate have an odor? Note both the color and odor if present. Has the patient noticed a change in either the characteristics or drainage of the lesion? If so, how and when?

From Thompson/Wilson.[24]

Types of Lesions

Primary skin lesions

Macule—Flat, nonpalpable, circumscribed, less than 1 cm in diameter, brown, red, purple, white, or tan

Patch—Flat, nonpalpable, irregularly shaped (macule greater than 1 cm in diameter)

Papule—Elevated, palpable, firm, circumscribed, less than 1 cm in diameter, brown, red, pink, tan, or bluish red

Plaque—Elevated, flat topped, firm, rough (superficial papule greater than 1 cm in diameter, may be coalesced papules)

Wheal—Elevated, irregularly shaped area of cutaneous edema, solid, transient, changing, variable diameter, pale pink

Nodule—Elevated, firm, circumscribed, palpable, deeper in dermis than papule, 1 to 2 cm in diameter

Tumor—Elevated, solid, may or may not be clearly demarcated, greater than 2 cm in diameter, may or may not vary from skin color

Vesicle—Elevated, circumscribed, superficial, filled with serous fluid, less than 1 cm in diameter

Bulla—Vesicle greater than 1 cm in diameter

Pustule—Elevated, superficial (similar to vesicle but filled with purulent fluid)

Cyst—Elevated, circumscribed, palpable, encapsulated, filled with liquid or semisolid material

Telangiectasia—Fine, irregular red line produced by dilation of capillary

Secondary skin lesions

Scale—Heaped-up keratinized cells, flaky exfoliation, irregular, thick or thin, dry or oily, varied size, silver, white, or tan

Crust—Dried serum, blood, or purulent exudate, slightly elevated, size varies, brown, red, black, tan, or straw

Lichenification—Rough, thickened epidermis, accentuated skin markings from rubbing or irritation, often involves flexor aspect of extremity

Scar—Thin to thick fibrous tissue replacing injured dermis, irregular, pink, red, or white, may be atrophic or hypertrophic

Keloid—Irregularly shaped, elevated, progressively enlarging scar, grows beyond boundaries of wound, from excessive collagen formation during healing

Excoriation—Loss of epidermis, linear of hollowed-out crusted area, dermis exposed

Fissure—Linear crack or break from epidermis to dermis, small, deep, red

Erosion—Loss of all or part of epidermis, depressed, moist, glistening (follows rupture of vesicle or bulla, larger than fissure)

Ulcer—Loss of epidermis and dermis, concave, size varies, exudative, red, or reddish blue

Atrophy—Thinning of skin surface and loss of skin markings, skin translucent and paperlike

Warning Signs for Changes in Moles and Other Pigmented Lesions

The following changes in skin moles or lesions are considered to be risk factors for carcinoma and require further medical investigation:

- A sudden enlargement or change in shape.
- Irregular borders of a mole that previously had a regular border.
- A change in color or variegated coloring.
- A mole or lesion that has maldistribution of color.
- Itching, tenderness, pain, or bleeding
- A change in surface characteristics, such as flaking, scaling, or oozing.
- A change in the surrounding skin, such as redness or swelling.

From Thompson/Wilson.24

GASTROINTESTINAL

Anatomic Correlates of the Nine Regions of the Abdomen

Right Hypochondriac	**Epigastric**	**Left Hypochondriac**
Right lobe of liver Gallbladder Portion of duodenum Hepatic flexure of colon Portion of right kidney Suprarenal gland	Pyloric end of stomach Duodenum Pancreas Portion of liver	Stomach Spleen Tail of pancreas Splenic flexure of colon Upper pole of left kidney Suprarenal gland
Right Lumbar	**Umbilical**	**Left Lumbar**
Ascending colon Lower half of right kidney Portion of duodenum and jejunum	Lower duodenum Jejunum and ileum	Descending colon Lower half of right kidney Portions of jejunum and ileum
Right Inguinal	**Hypogastric**	**Left Inguinal**
Cecum Appendix Ileum (lower end) Right ureter Right spermatic cord Right ovary	Ileum Bladder Uterus (in pregnancy)	Sigmoid colon Left ureter Left spermatic cord Left ovary

From Thompson/Wilson.[24]

Phases of HIV Infection and AIDS

Phase	Length of phase	Antibodies detectable	Symptoms	Can be transmitted
1. Window period	4 wk to 6 mo after infection	No	None	Yes
2. Acute primary HIV infection	1-2 wk	Possible	Flu-like illness	Yes
3. Asymptomatic infection	1-15 or more yr	Yes	None	Yes
4. Symptomatic immune suppression	Up to 3 yr	Yes	Fever, night sweats, weight loss, diarrhea, neuropathy, fatigue, rashes, lymphadenopathy, cognitive slowing, oral lesions	Yes
5. AIDS	Variable: 1-5 yr from first AIDS-defining condition	Yes	Severe opportunistic infections and tumors in any body system; neurologic manifestations	Yes

From Grimes.[13]

Staging System of Kaposi's Sarcoma

Stage	Description
I	Cutaneous, locally indolent
II	Cutaneous, locally aggressive with or without regional lymph nodes
III	Generalized mucocutaneous or lymph node involvement
IV	Visceral
Subtypes	
A. No systemic signs or symptoms	
B. Systemic signs: 10% weight loss or temperature greater than 100°F orally, unrelated to identifiable source of infection, and lasting more than 2 weeks	
Generalized: more than upper or lower extremities alone; includes minimal gastrointestinal disease defined as more than five lesions and larger than 2 cm in combined diameters	

INFECTION

Body Substance Isolation

1. *All* health care workers should use appropriate barrier precautions to prevent skin and mucous membrane exposure when contact with blood or body fluids of *any* patient is anticipated.
2. Gloves should be worn for touching blood and body fluids, mucous membranes, or nonintact skin of all patients, for handling items or surfaces soiled with blood or body fluids, and for performing venipuncture and other vascular access procedures. Gloves should be changed after contact with each patient.
3. Hands and other skin surfaces should be washed immediately and thoroughly if contaminated with blood or other body fluids. Hands should be washed immediately after gloves are removed.
4. Masks and protective eyewear or face shields should be worn during procedures that are likely to generate droplets of blood or other body fluids.
5. Gowns or aprons should be worn during procedures that are likely to generate splashes of blood or other body fluids.
6. Needles should not be recapped, purposely bent or broken by hand, removed from disposable syringes, or otherwise manipulated by hand. After use, disposable syringes and needles, scalpel blades, and other sharp items should be placed in puncture-resistant containers for disposal; the containers should be located as close as practical to the use area. Large-bore reusable needles should be placed in a puncture-resistant container for transport to the reprocessing area.
7. Although saliva has not been implicated in HIV transmission, mouthpieces, resuscitation bags, or other ventilation devices should be available for use in areas in which the need for resuscitation is predictable.

8. Health care workers who have exudative lesions or weeping dermatitis should refrain from all direct patient care and from handling patient care equipment until the condition resolves.
9. Pregnant health care workers are not known to be at greater risk of contracting HIV infection than nonpregnant workers; however, if a pregnant worker develops HIV infection, the infant is at risk from perinatal transmission. Pregnant health care workers should strictly adhere to precautions.
10. Invasive procedures (surgical entry into tissues, cavities, or organs) or repair of major traumatic injuries carries a risk of splattering of blood and fluids and requires the use of gloves, masks, protective eyewear or face shield, and gowns or aprons made of materials that provide an effective fluid barrier.
11. During an invasive procedure, if a glove is torn or a needlestick or other injury occurs, the glove should be removed and a new glove used as promptly as patient safety permits; the needle or instrument involved in the incident should be removed from the sterile field.

From Centers for Disease Control.[8]

Notifiable Diseases in the United States

AIDS
Amebiasis*
Anthrax
Aseptic meningitis*
Botulism†
Brucellosis
Chancroid†
Cholera
Diphtheria
Encephalitis, primary*
Encephalitis, postinfectious*
Escherichia coli O157:H7†
Gonorrhea
Granuloma inguinale*
Haemophilus influenzae, invasive
Hansen disease (leprosy)
Hepatitis A
Hepatitis B
Hepatitis, non-A, non-B
Hepatitis C, unspecified*
Legionellosis
Leptospirosis*
Lyme disease
Lymphogranuloma venereum*
Malaria
Measles
Meningococcal disease
Mumps
Pertussis
Plague
Poliomyelitis
Psittacosis
Rabies, animal
Rabies, human
Rheumatic fever*
Rocky Mountain spotted fever (RMSF)
Rubella
Rubella, congenital syndrome
Salmonellosis†
Shigellosis†
Syphilis
Syphilis, congenital
Tetanus
Toxic-shock syndrome
Trichinosis
Tuberculosis
Tularemia*
Typhoid fever
Yellow fever†

---

*Deleted from the nationally notifiable disease list in 1995.
†Not published in the weekly tables.

Recommended Immunization Schedule—Infants and Children Born in United States

Recommended Age[b]	Immunization(s)[c]	Comments
Birth	HBV[d]	
1-2 months	HBV[d]	
2 months	DTP, Hib, OPV	DTP and OPV can be initiated as early as 4 weeks after birth in areas of high endemicity or during outbreaks
4 months	DTP, Hib, OPV	2-month interval (minimum of 6 weeks) recommended for OPV
6 months	DTP, (Hib[c])	
6-18 months	HBV,[d] OPV	
12-15 months	Hib, MMR	MMR should be given at 12 months of age in high-risk areas; if indicated, tuberculin testing may be done at the same visit
15-18 months	DTaP or DTP	The fourth dose of diphtheria-tetanus-pertussis vaccine should be given 6 to 12 months after the third dose of DTP and may be given as early as 12 months of age, provided that the interval between doses 3 and 4 is at least 6 months and DTP is given; DTaP is not currently licensed for use in children younger than 15 months
4-6 years	DTaP or DTP, OPV	DTaP or DTP and OPV should be given at or before school entry; DTP or DTaP should not be given at or after the seventh birthday

Recommended Age[b]	Immunization(s)[c]	Comments
11-12 years	MMR	MMR should be given at entry to middle school or junior high school unless two doses were given after the first birthday
14-16 years	Td	Repeat every 10 years throughout life

Modified from American Academy of Pediatrics, Committee on Infectious Diseases: 1994 Red Book: Report of the Committee on Infectious Diseases, *ed 23, Elk Grove Village, IL, 1994, The Academy.*

[a]*Table is not completely consistent with all package inserts. For products used, also consult manufacturer's package insert for instructions on storage, handling, dosage, and administration. Biologics prepared by different manufacturers may vary, and package inserts of the same manufacturer may change from time to time. Therefore the practitioner should be aware of the contents of the current package insert.*

[b]*These recommended ages should not be construed as absolute. For example, 2 months can be 6 to 10 weeks. However, MMR usually should not be given to children younger than 12 months. If measles vaccination is indicated, monovalent measles vaccine is recommended, and MMR should be given subsequently at 12 to 15 months.*

[c]*Vaccine abbreviations:* HBV, *hepatitis B virus vaccine;* DTP, *diphtheria and tetanus toxoids and pertussis vaccine;* DTaP, *diphtheria and tetanus toxoids and acellular pertussis vaccine;*Hib, Haemophilus influenzae *type b conjugate vaccine;* OPV, *oral poliovirus vaccine (containing attenuated poliovirus types 1, 2, and 3);* MMR, *live measles, mumps, and rubella viruses vaccine;* Td, *adult tetanus toxoid (full dose) and diphtheria toxoid (reduced dose), for children ≥7 years and adults.*

[d]*An acceptable alternative to minimize number of visits for immunizing infants of HBsAg-negative mothers is to administer dose 1 at 0-2 months, dose 2-4 months, and dose 3 at 6-18 months.*

[e]*Hib; dose 3 of Hib is not indicated if the product for doses 1 and 2 was PedvaxHIB (PRP-OMP).*

	Staphylococcal food poisoning	Botulism
Reservoir	Humans; cows with infected udders; dogs and fowl	Soil, water, and intestinal tract of animals and fish
Transmission	Ingestion of food containing staphylococcal toxin, which formed while food was held at room temperature	Ingestion of food in which toxin has formed; generally home-canned vegetables, fruits, and meats; also onions and potatoes cooked and held at room temperature
Incubation period	30 min-7 h, usually 2-4 h	12-36 h

From Grimes.[13]

Food Poisoning: Enteric Infections

	Clostridium perfringens	*Vibrio parahaemolyticus*	*Bacillus cereus*
Reservoir	Soil and gastrointestinal tract of humans and animals	Marine silt, coastal waters, fish, and shellfish	Soil; commonly found in raw, dried, and processed foods
Transmission	Ingestion of food, especially meat, contaminated by soil or feces; spores survive normal cooking temperatures, germinate, and multiply during cooking and reheating	Ingestion of raw or undercooked contaminated seafood; food contaminated with seawater	Ingestion of food that has been kept at ambient temperatures after cooking, permitting multiplication of the organism
Incubation period	6-24 h; usually 10-12 h	4-96 h; usually 12-24 h	1-6 h for disease causing vomiting; 6-20 h for disease causing diarrhea

From Grimes.[13]

Childhood Communicable and Immunizable Infectious Diseases

	Chickenpox	Tetanus	Diphtheria	Pertussis (whooping cough)
Transmission	Direct and indirect contact with droplets from respiratory passages; an extremely contagious disease	Tetanus spores enter body through a wound contaminated with soil and feces; necrotic tissue favors the growth of the bacillus	Direct or indirect contact with exudate from mucous membranes of infected person or carrier; raw milk may also be a vehicle	Direct contact with droplets from respiratory passages
Incubation period	2-3 wk; commonly 13-17 days	3-21 days; commonly 10 days	2-5 days	7-21 days; commonly 7 days
Report to local health authority	In some areas	Case report required	Case report required	Case report required

	Poliomyelitis	Mumps (infectious parotiditis)	Rubella (German measles)	Rubeola (hard measles)
Transmission	Direct and indirect contact with respiratory discharges and feces; fecal-oral route more common than respiratory transmission	Direct contact with saliva droplets from infected person	Direct or indirect contact with nasopharyngeal sections of infected persons; transplacental transmission leads to congenital rubella syndrome	Direct or indirect contact with nasal secretions from infected persons; highly communicable
Incubation period	3-35 days; commonly 7-14 days	2-3 wk; commonly 18 days	14-23 days; commonly 16-18 days	Commonly 10 days; 8-13 days until fever; 14 days until rash
Report to local health authority	Case report required	Case report required in some areas	Case report required	Case report required

From Benenson.[5]

CANCER
Risk Factors for Cancer

Cervical Cancer

- Onset of intercourse before the age of 20
- Multiple sex partners
- Infections with human papilloma virus (HPV)
- Cigarette smoking
- Lower socioeconomic status
- Age between 40 and 50 years

Ovarian Cancer

- Age 50 or older
- Family history of ovarian cancer
- More than 40 years of active ovulation
- Nulliparity or first pregnancy after age 30
- High-fat, low-fiber diet; vitamin A-deficient diet
- Prolonged exposure to asbestos and talc

Endometrial Cancer

- Large body frame and obesity
- High-fat diet
- Nulliparity
- Infertility
- Menstrual irregularities
- Late onset of menopause
- Dysfunctional uterine bleeding during menopause
- Adenomatous hyperplasia of the endometrium
- Family history of breast, colon, or ovarian cancer

- History of diabetes or hypertension
- Family history of endocrine cancers

Breast Cancer

- Age 40 years or older (80% of all breast cancer)
- Female
- Female family member with breast cancer history
- Menarche before 12 years of age
- Menopause after 55 years of age
- Has never given birth to a child
- Had first child after 30 years of age
- Previous personal history of any type of cancer

Colorectal Cancer

- Over 40 years of age (peak ages 65-74)
- Family history of colon cancer, familial polyposis, Gardner syndrome, Peutz-Jeghers syndrome
- Personal history of colon polyps; Crohn's disease; Gardner syndrome; ovarian, breast, or endometrial cancer; ulcerative colitis of more than 10 year's duration
- Diet high in beef and animal fats, low in fiber
- Exposure to asbestos, acrylics, and other carcinogens

From Seidel.[20]

Tumor Classification

T	**Primary tumor classification by depth of invasion, surface spread, and size**
T0	No evidence of a primary lesion
T1	Superficial lesion confined to organ of origin
T2	Localized lesion with deep invasion into adjacent structure
T3	Advanced lesion confined to an anatomic region of organ of origin
T4	Advanced lesion extending into adjacent organs
N	**Lymph node involvement**
N0	No evidence of disease
N1	Palpable, movable nodes limited to primary site
N2, N3, N4	Progressive increase in size, fixation, and location of palpable nodes
M	**Anatomic extent of metastasis**
M0	NO metastasis
M1	Isolated metastasis confined to one organ or site
M2	Multiple metastases confined to one organ or site; no functional impairment
M3	Multiple organs involved; minimal functional impairment
M4	Multiple organ involvement; significant functional impairment

From Beare, Myers.[4]

SECTION II DRUGS

DRUG DOSAGE FORMULA

Use the following formulas for quick calculation of drug dosages.

Drug volume to be administered

$$(\text{ml}) = \frac{\text{Desired dose (mg)}}{\text{Drug concentration (mg/ml)}}$$

$$\textit{or} = \frac{\text{Desired dose (mg)} \times \text{volume (ml)}}{\text{Amount (mg)}}$$

NOTE: drug concentration (mg/ml) $= \frac{\text{Amount (mg)}}{\text{Volume (ml)}}$

From Madigan.[14]

IV FLOW RATE FORMULA

Use the following formulas to calculate IV flow rates.

$$\text{Flow rate (ml/hr)} = \frac{\text{Desired dose (mg/min)} \times 60 \text{ (min/hr)}}{\text{Drug concentration (mg/ml)}}$$

$$or = \frac{\text{Desired dose } (\mu\text{g/kg/min}) \times 60\text{(min/hr)} \times \text{wt } (kg)}{\text{Drug concentration } (\mu\text{g/ml})}$$

$$or = \frac{\text{Drip rate (drops/min)} \times 60 \text{ (min/hr)}}{60 \text{ (drops/ml)}}$$

$$\text{Drip rate (drops/min)} = \frac{\text{Total volume to be infused (ml)} \times \text{drop factor (drops/ml)}}{\text{Total time for the infusion (min)}}$$

$$or = \frac{\text{Drops/ml}}{60 \text{ (min/hr)}} \times \frac{\text{Volume to be infused (ml/hr)}}{1}$$

SECTION III

NORMAL LABORATORY VALUES, CAUSES, FORMULAS, AND CONVERSIONS

Test	Values	Abnormal Findings	
Serum Chemistry			
Bilirubin (Bil)			
Adult/elderly/child		**Increased Levels**	
Total	0.1-1.0 mg/dl	Dubin-Johnson syndrome	
Indirect	0.2-0.8 mg/dl	Erythroblastosis fetalis	
Direct	0.1-0.3 mg/dl	Cirrhosis	
Newborn		Hepatitis	
Total	1-12 mg/dl	Large-volume blood transfusions	
		Bile duct obstruction	
		Pernicious anemia	
		Sickle cell anemia	
		Transfusion reaction	
Creatinine (Creat)		**Increased Levels**	**Decreased levels**
Adult: female	0.5-1.1 mg/dl	Glomerulonephritis	Debilitation
male	0.6-1.2	Pyelonephritis	Decreased muscle mass

Test	Values	Abnormal Findings	
Creatinine (Creat) (cont'd)			
Adolescent	0.5-1.0 mg/dl	Acute tubular necrosis	
Child	0.3-0.7 mg/dl	Decreased renal blood flow	
Infant	0.2-0.4 mg/dl	Diabetes	
Newborn	0.3-1.2 mg/dl	Nephritis	
Urea Nitrogen (BUN)		**Increased levels**	**Decreased levels**
Adult	10-20 mg/dl	Renal disease	Liver failure
Child	5-18 mg/dl	Urinary obstruction	Overhydration
Infant	5-18 mg/dl	Hypovolemia	Negative nitrogen balance
Newborn	3-12 mg/dl	Myocardial infarction	Pregnancy
		Congestive heart failure	
		Gastrointestinal bleeding	
		Renal failure	
		Dehydration	

Test	Values	Abnormal Findings	
Glucose (fasting)[FBS]		**Increased (hyperglycemia)**	**Decreased (hypoglycemia)**
Critical values		Diabetes mellitus	Insulinoma
Adult male	<50 and >400 mg/dl	Acute stress response	Hypothyroidism
Adult female	<40 and >400 mg/dl	Cushing's disease	Hypopituitarism
		Hyperparathyroidism	Addison's disease
Normal values			
Infant	40-90 mg/dl		
Child	60-105 mg/dl		
Electrolytes		**Increased (hyperkalemia)**	**Decreased (hypokalemia)**
Potassium (K+)			
Adults	3.5-5.0 mEq/L	Increased potassium intake	Decreased potassium intake
Child	3.4-4.7 mEq/L	Renal failure	Gastrointestinal disorders
Infant	4.1-5.3 mEq/L	Addison's disease	Diuretics

Test	Values	Abnormal Findings	
Potassium (cont'd)			
Newborn	3.9-5.9 mEq/L	Hypoaldosteronism Acidosis Infection Transfusion of hemolyzed blood	Hyperaldosteronism Cushing's syndrome Alkalosis Insulin or glucose administration
Sodium (Na+)		**Increased (hypernatremia)**	**Decreased (hyponatremia)**
Adults	136-145 mEq/L	Increased sodium intake	Decreased sodium intake
Child	136-145 mEq/L	Decreased sodium loss	Addison's disease
Infant	134-150 mEq/L	Excessive sweating	Diarrhea

Test	Values	Abnormal Findings	
Sodium—(cont'd)			
		Increased (hypernatremia)	**Decreased (hyponatremia)**
Newborn	134-144 mEq/L	Diabetes insipidus Extensive thermal burns Osmotic diuresis	Vomiting or nasogastric aspiration Diuretic administration Excessive oral or IV intake Ascites Congestive heart failure
Clorides (Cl^-)		**Increased (hyperchloremia)**	**Decreased (hypochloremia)**
Adult			
Child	90-110 mEq/L 90-110 mEq/L	Dehydration Renal tubular acidosis	Overhydration Congestive heart failiure

Test	Values	Abnormal Findings	
Newborn	96-106 mEq/L	Cushing's syndrome Eclampsia Multiple myeloma Kidney dysfunction Metabolic acidosis Hyperventilation	Vomiting Gastric suctioning Chronic respiratory acidosis Addison's disease Burns Metabolic alkalosis Hypokalemia
Carbon dioxide (CO_2)		**Increased**	**Decreased**
Adult	23-30 mEq/L	Severe vomiting	Severe diarrhea
Child	20-28 mEq/L	Aldosteronism	Starvation
Infant	20-28 mEq/L	Emphysema	
Newborn	13-22 mEq/L	Metabolic alkalosis Gastric suctioning Renal failure Diabetic ketoacidosis Metabolic acidosis Shock	

Test	Values	Abnormal Findings	
Serum Enzymes			
Amylase			
Normal	56-190 IU/L	**Increased**	
		Acute pancreatitis	Necrotic bowel
		Perforated peptic ulcer	Acute cholecystitis
		Perforated bowel	Ectopic pregnancy
		Parotiditis (mumps)	
		Pulmonary infarction	Diabetic ketoacidosis
Creatinine phosphokinase (CPK)		**Increased total**	
Adult: male	12-70 U/ml	Acute myocardial infarction	Pulmonary infarction
Adult: female	10-55 U/ml	Convulsions	Dermatomyositis
		Muscular dystrophy	Chronic alcoholism
		Hypokalemia	
Lactic dehydrogenase (LDH)		**Increased**	
Adult	45-90 U/L	Myocardial infarction	Renal parenchymal diseases

Test	Values	Abnormal Findings	
Lactic dehydrogenase (cont'd)		**Increased**	
Child		Pulmonary diseases	Intestinal ischemia
Infant	60-170 U/L	Hepatic diseases	Skeletal muscle diseases
Newborn	100-250 U/L	Red blood cell diseases	Cerebral vascular accident
	160-450 U/L	Infectious mononucleosis	Pancreatitis
			Collagen diseases
		Heat stroke	Hypotension
		Muscular dystrophy	
Alanine aminotransaminase (SGPT)		**Increased**	
Adult/child	5-35 IU/L	Hepatitis	Hepatic ischemia
		Cirrhosis	Hepatic tumor
		Hepatic necrosis	Hepatotoxic drugs
		Cholestasis	

Test	Values	Abnormal Findings	
Aspartate aminotransaminase (SGOT)			
Adult/child	8-20 U/L or 5-40 IU/L	**Increased**	**Decreased**
		Myocardial infarction	Diabetic Ketoacidosis
		Increased	**Decreased**
Newborn	15-60 U/L	Hepatitis	Pregnancy
		Hepatic pancreatitis	Beriberi
		Skeletal muscle trauma	
		Multiple trauma	
		Hepatic necrosis	
		Acute hemolytic anemia	
		Primary muscle diseases	
Hematology			
Coagulation			
Bleeding time		**Prolonged time**	
Normal	1-9 minutes	Bone marrow failure	

Test	Values	Abnormal Findings
Critical value	>12 minutes	Primary or metastic tumor infiltrating bone marrow Disseminated intravascular coagulation (DIC) Thrombocytopenia Collagen vascular diseases Clotting factor deficiencies Hemophilia Leukemia
Partial thromboplastin time (PTT) Normal	60-70 seconds	**Increased** Clotting factor deficiencies **Decreased** Early stages of DIC

Test	Values	Abnormal Findings	
Bleeding time—cont'd			
Critical value	>100 seconds	Cirrhosis of the liver Vitamin K deficiency Leukemia DIC Heparin administration Hemophilia	Extensive cancer
Prothrombin time (PT)		**Increased**	
Normal	11-12.5 seconds	Cirrhosis of the liver	Bile duct obstruction
Critical value	> 20 seconds	Hepatitis Vitamin K deficiency	DIC Salicylate intoxication
Hematocrit (Hct)		**Increased**	**Decreased**
Male	42%-52%	Congenital heart disease	Anemia
Female	37%-47%	Polycythemia vera	Hyperthyroidism
Child	31%-43%	Severe dehydration	Cirrhosis
Infant	30%-40%	Shock	Hemolytic reaction

Test	Values	Abnormal Findings	
Hematocrit (Hct) (cont'd)			
Newborn	44%-64%	Erythrocytosis Severe diarrhea Eclampsia Trauma Burns Dehydration	Hemorrhage Dietary deficiency Hodgkin's disease Normal pregnancy Rheumatoid arthritis Malnutrition Leukemias
Hemoglobin (Hb,Hgb)		**Increased**	**Decreased**
Male	14-18 g/dl	Congenital heart disease	Anemia Severe hemorrhage
Female	12-16 g/dl	Polycythemia vera	
Child	11-16 g/dl	Hemoconcentration of blood	Hemolysis Hodgkin's disease
Infant	10-15 g/dl	COPD	

Test	Values	Abnormal Findings	
Hemoglobin cont'd			
Newborn	14-24 g/dl	Congestive heart failure High altitudes Severe burns Dehydration	Sickle cell anemia Cancer Nutritional deficiency Lymphoma Kidney diseases Chronic hemorrhage
Erythrocyte sedimentation rate (ESR, Sed rate)		**Increased**	**Decreased**
Male	up to 15 mm/hr	Toxemia	Congestive heart failure
Female	up to 20 mm/hr	Nephritis	Sickle cell anemia
Child	up to 10 mm/hr	Multiple myeloma	Hypofibrinogenemia

Test	Values	Abnormal Findings	
Newborn	0-2 mm/hr	Bacterial infections Acute pelvic inflammatory disease Pneumonia Rheumatoid arthritis Rheumatic fever Myocardial infarction	Polycythemia vera Infectious mononucleosis Degenerative arthritis Angina pectoris
White blood cell count (WBC)			
Total WBCs			
Adult/child > 2 yrs	5000-10,000/mm^3		
Child 2 yrs and <	6200-17,000/mm^3		
Newborn	9000-30,000/mm^3		

Test	Values	Abnormal Findings	
Differential count		**Increased (neutrophilia)**	**Decreased (neutropenia)**
Neutrophils	55%-70%	Physical/emotional stress Acute infection Myelocytic leukemia Trauma Inflamatory diseases Metabolic disorders	Aplastic anemia Dietary deficiency Overwhelming infection Viral infections Radiation therapy Chemotherapy
Lymphocytes	20%-40%	**Increased (lymphocytosis)** Chronic bacterial infection Viral infection Lymphocytic leukemia Multiple myeloma Infectious mononucleosis Infectious hepatitis	**Decreased (lymphocytopenia)** Leukemia Sepsis Immunodeficiency diseases Late stages of HIV Lupus erythematosus Drug therapy

Test	Values	Abnormal Findings	
Monocytes	2%-8%	**Increased (monocytosis)** Chronic inflammatory disease Viral infections Tuberculosis Chronic ulcerative colitis Parasites (e.g., malaria)	**Decreased (monocytopenia)** Drug therapy: prednisone
Eosinophilis	1%-4%	**Increased (eosinophilia)** Parasitic infections Allergic reactions Eczema Leukemia Autoimmune disease	**Decreased (eosinopenia)** Increased adrenosteroid production

Test	Values	Abnormal Findings	
Differential count—cont'd		**Increased (basophilia)**	**Decreased (basopenia)**
Basophils	0.5%-1%	Myelofibrosis Polycythemia rubra vera Leukemia	Acute allergic reaction Hyperthyroidism Stress reaction

CALCULATION FORMULAS AND NORMAL RANGES

Parameter	Formula	Normal range
Cardiac output (CO)	$HR \times SV$	4-8 L/min
Cardiac index (CI)	$\frac{CO}{BSA}$	2.8-4.2 L/min/m^2
Stroke volume (SV)	$\frac{CO \times 1000}{HR}$	60-130 ml/beat
Stroke volume index (SVI)	$\frac{SV}{BSA}$	33-75 ml/m^2/beat
Stroke index (SI)	$\frac{CI}{HR} \times 1000$	30-65 ml/m^2/beat
Mean arterial pressure (MAP)	$\frac{2(DBP) + SBP}{3}$	70-105 mm Hg
Coronary perfusion pressure (CPP)	Arterial DP – PAWP	60-80 mm Hg
Systemic vascular resistance (SVR)	$\frac{MAP - CVP}{CO} \times 80$	700-1600 dynes/sec/cm^{-5}
Pulmonary vascular resistance (PRV)	$\frac{PAM - PAWP}{CO} \times 80$	20-130 dynes/sec/cm^{-5}

Parameter	Formula	Normal range
Left ventricular stroke work index (LVSWI)	(MAP – PAWP)SVI $\times$ 0.136	35-85 g/m^2/beat
Right ventricular stroke work index (RVSWI)	(PAM – CVP)SVI $\times$ 0.136	8.5-12 g/m^2/beat
Ejection fraction (EF)	$\frac{SV}{\text{end diastolic volume}} \times 100$	60%
Rate pressure product (RPP)	HR $\times$ SBP	<12,000
Arterial oxygen content (CaO_2)	(SaO_2 $\times$ Hb $\times$ 1.38) + (PaO_2 $\times$ .0031)	18-20 ml/100 ml or 20 vol %
Venous oxygen content (CvO_2)	(SvO_2 $\times$ Hb $\times$ 1.38) + (PvO_2 $\times$ .0031)	15.5 ml/100 ml
Arterial venous oxygen content difference ($C_{(a-v)}O_2$)	$CaO_2 - CvO_2$	4-6 ml/100 ml
Arterial oxygen delivery (DO_2)	CO $\times$ 10 $\times$ CaO_2	900-1200 ml/min
Venous oxygen delivery (DO_2)	CO $\times$ 10 $\times$ CvO_2	775 ml/min
Oxygen consumption (VO_2)	CO $\times$ 10 $\times$ $_{(a-v)}O_2$	200-250 ml/min

CALCULATION FORMULAS AND NORMAL RANGES—cont'd

Parameter	Formula	Normal range
Mixed venous oxygen saturation (SvO_2)	$1-VO_2/DO_2$	60%-80%
Alveolar-arterial oxygen gradient ($AaDO_2$)	$PAO_2 - PaO_2$	< 15 mm Hg
Alveolar partial pressure of oxygen (PaO_2)	$FIO_2 - Paco_2/0.8$	
Respiratory quotient (RQ)	$\frac{O_2 \text{ consumption}}{CO_2 \text{ production}}$	0.8-1
Neurologic		
Cerebral perfusion pressure (CPP)	MPA – ICP	80-100 mm Hg
Intracranial pressure (ICP)		0-15 mm Hg
Renal		
Anion gap (GAP)	$Na - (HCO_3 + Cl)$	8-16 mEq/L
Osmolality (OSM)	(2Na) + K + BUN/3 + Glucose/18	275-295 mOsm
Glomerular filtration rate (GRF)	$\frac{(140 - \text{Age}) \times \text{wt (kg)}}{\text{(male) } 75 \times \text{serum Cr}}$ (female) 85 × serum Cr	80-120 ml/min

From Stillwell.[23]

Miscellaneous Calculations

$\mu g/ml = mg/ml \times 1000$

$ml/min = ml/hr \div 60$

$$\mu g/kg/min = \frac{\mu g/ml \times ml/min}{wt\ (kg)}$$

$$ml/hr = \frac{wt(kg) \times \mu g/kg/min}{\mu/ml} \times 60$$

Conversion Factors

1 kg	= 1 liter fluid	1/150 gr	= 0.4 mg
1 mg	= 1000 μg	1 tsp	= 5 ml
1 kg	= 2.2 lb	1 Tbsp	= 15 ml
1 gr	= 60 mg	1 oz	= 30 ml
1/100 gr	= 0.6 mg	1 mm Hg	= 1.36 cm H_2O

From Stillwell.[23]

Equivalents and Conversions

Liquid Volume

Apothecary (household)	Approximate metric (ml)
1 gallon (gal)	4000
1 quart (qt)	1000
1 pint (pt)	500
½ pint	250
1 cup	240
1 ounce (oz)	30
1 tablespoon (Tbsp)	15
1 teaspoon (tsp)	5

Weights

Apothecary (household)	Approximate metric
2.2 pounds (lb)	1 kg
1 pound	500 g
1 ounce (oz)	30 g
15 grains (gr)	1 g
1 grain	60 mg

Pressures	Miscellaneous
14.7 psi = 1 atm = 760 torr = 760 mm Hg	1 ml = 1 cc
1 psi = 6.9 kPa	IV Tubing
1 kPa = 0.15 psi	1 ml = 60 microdrops
1 cm H_2O = 1.36 mm Hg	1 ml = 20, 15, or 10 macrodrops (depends on the manufacturer)
1 mm Hg = 0.74 cm H_2O	°C = (°F − 32) × 5/9
	°F = (°C × 9/5) + 32
	1 Joule (J) = 1 watt-second (w-s)

From Madigan.[14]

REFERENCES

1. Agency for Health Care Policy and Research: Clinical Practice Guidelines: Acute Pain Management: *Operative or Medical Procedures and Trauma,* Rockville, Maryland, 1992, U.S. Department of Health and Human Services, Public Health Service.
2. American Heart Association: Standards and guidelines for cardiopulmonary resuscitation and emergency cardiac care, *JAMA* 225:2841, 1986.
3. American Nurses Association: *Standards of clinical nursing practice,* Washington, DC, 1991, The Association.
4. Beare PG, Myers JL: *Principles and practice of adult health nursing,* ed 2, St Louis, 1994, Mosby.
5. Benenson A, editor: *Control of communicable diseases in man,* ed 14, Washington, DC, 1985, American Public Health Association.
6. Brunner LS, Suddarth DS: *Textbook of medical-surgical nursing,* ed 6, Philadelphia, 1988, JB Lippincott.
7. Canobbio M: *Cardiovascular disorders,* St Louis, 1990, Mosby.
8. Centers for Disease Control: Recommendations for prevention of HIV transmission in health-care settings, *MMWR* 36(suppl 2), 1987.
9. Centers for Disease Control: Recommendations of the Immunization Practices Advisory Committee: general recommendations on immunization, *MMWR* 39(13):205, 1989.
10. Centers for Disease Control: Recommendations of the Immunization Practices Advisory Committee: *Haemophilus* B conjugate vaccines for prevention of *Haemophilus influenzae* type b disease among infants and children 2 months of age and older, *MMWR* 40(RR-1), 1991.

11. Centers for Disease Control: Summary of notifiable diseases, United States, 1989, *MMWR* 38(54), Oct 5, 1990.
12. Chipps E, Clanin N, Campbell V: *Neurological disorders,* St Louis, 1992, Mosby.
13. Grimes DE: *Infectious diseases,* St Louis, 1991, Mosby.
14. Madigan KG: *Prehospital emergency drugs: pocket reference,* St Louis, 1990, Mosby.
15. McCaffery M, Beebe A: *Pain: clinical manual for nursing practice,* St Louis, 1989, Mosby.
16. Mourad LA: *Orthopedic disorders,* St Louis, 1991, Mosby.
17. Otto SE: *Oncology nursing,* St Louis, 1997, Mosby.
18. Pagana KD, Pagana TJ: *Mosby's diagnostic and laboratory test reference,* ed 2, St Louis, 1995, Mosby.
19. Seidel et al: *Mosby's guide to physical examination,* ed 3, St Louis, 1995, Mosby.
20. Seeley, RR, Stephens TD, Tate P: *Anatomy and Physiology,* ed 3, St Louis, 1995, Mosby.
21. Sheehy SB, Lombardi JE: *Manual of emergency care,* ed 4, St Louis, 1995, Mosby.
22. Stillwell SB: *Quick critical care reference,* ed 2, St Louis, 1994, Mosby.
23. Thompson JM, Wilson SF: *Health assessment for nursing practice,* St Louis, 1996, Mosby.
24. Wilson SF, Thompson JM: *Respiratory disorders,* St Louis, 1991, Mosby.
25. Wong DL: *Pediatric quick reference,* ed 2, St Louis, 1995, Mosby.

NOTES

NOTES

NOTES

NOTES

NOTES

NOTES

NOTES

NOTES

NOTES

NOTES

NOTES